HERBAL REMEDIES THAT CURE ALL DISEASES

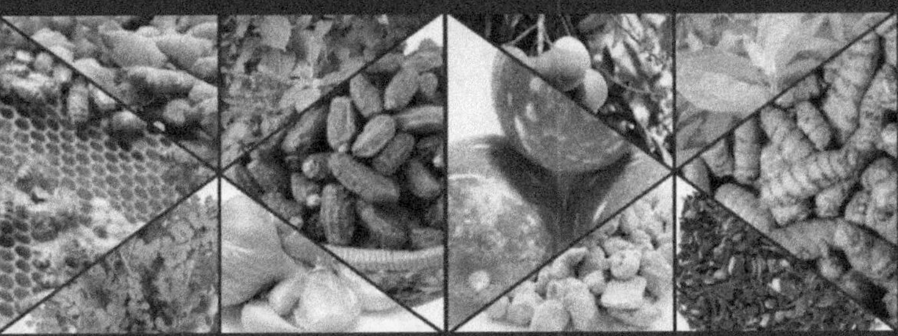

volume one

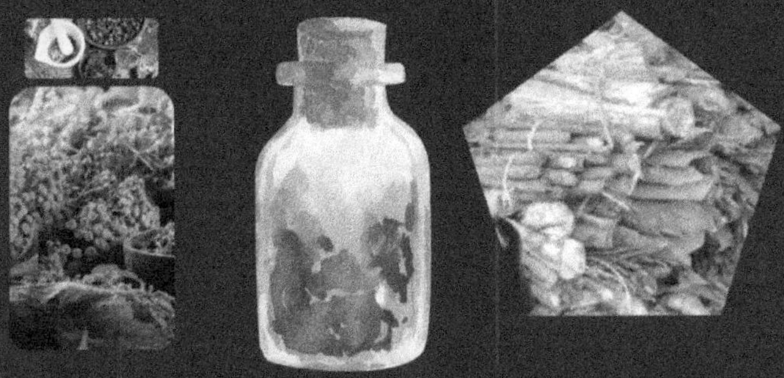

Gabriel Olatuja

HERBAL REMEDIES THAT CURE ALL DISEASES

VOLUME 1

Apostle Gabriel Olatuja

Contact the author through
gabrielolatuja@gmail.com,
olatujagabriel@gmail.com, or Call/WhatsApp
+2348067380225 or visit
www.gabrielolatuja.com.ng.

Gabriel-Wealth Olatuja Publishers

I am grateful to God for the grace he has given me, because no one receive anything, except it is given by our God. (John 3:27)

THE USE OF ROOT AND HERBS OR MEDICATIONS IS BIBLICAL

For those who think the use of herbal medications or medical treatment is a sin, I want to let you know that it is not. God gave us plants, animals for us to use as food and for our healthy living.

In Genesis 1:29, *Then God said, "Behold, I have given you every plant yielding seed that is on the surface of all the earth, and every tree which has fruit yielding seed; it shall be food for you"*

Genesis 9:3, *"Every moving thing that is alive shall be food for you; I give all to you, as I gave the green plant."*

Genesis 1:11, *Then God said, "Let the earth sprout vegetation, plants yielding seed, and fruit trees on the earth bearing fruit after their kind with seed in them"; and it was so."*

Psalm 104:14, *"He causes the grass to grow for the cattle, And vegetation for the labor of man, So that he may bring forth food from the earth"*

Genesis 1:12, *"The earth brought forth vegetation, plants yielding seed after their kind, and trees bearing fruit with seed in them, after their kind; and God saw that it was good."*

God created a diverse array of plants and animals, each containing unique nutritional benefits intended to promote vitality, healing, and bolster our immune systems. These natural provisions serve as a gift to humanity, offering nourishment and support for our physical well-being. Furthermore, through the advancements of medical science, many of these plants and animals have been transformed into medications, allowing for faster health outcomes and precise dosages.

Therefore, the utilization of roots, herbs, and medications derived from plants and animals is not considered a sin. Instead, it is a recognition of the bountiful resources provided by the Creator for the betterment of human health and well-being. As stewards of these gifts, it is our responsibility to utilize them wisely and in accordance with sound medical advice, ensuring optimal health outcomes and reverence for the blessings bestowed upon us.

WHAT INSPIRED THIS BOOK

"Herbal Remedies that Cure all Diseases" didn't just spring from one single source of inspiration, but rather from a confluence of experiences, observations, and passions. The seed for this book was planted in the fertile soil of a personal journey towards holistic health and a deep-seated curiosity about the healing power of nature.

First and foremost, the inspiration stemmed from a desire to explore alternatives to conventional medicine. In an age where synthetic drugs often come with a myriad of side effects and risks, there's a growing interest in returning to natural remedies that have been used for centuries. This book was born from a conviction that the earth offers an abundance of healing plants, waiting to be rediscovered and harnessed for their medicinal properties.

The author's own encounters with traditional herbal medicine played a significant role in shaping the book's direction. Whether it was witnessing the soothing effects of chamomile tea on a troubled stomach or marveling at the potency of garlic as a natural antibiotic, these personal experiences underscored the potential of herbs to heal a wide range of ailments.

Moreover, the author was inspired by the wisdom of ancient cultures that have long relied on herbal remedies to treat illness and promote wellness. From Ayurveda in India to Traditional Chinese Medicine, indigenous healing traditions around the world offer a wealth of knowledge about the therapeutic properties of plants. "Herbal Remedies that Cure all Diseases" draws from this rich tapestry of wisdom, weaving together age-old practices with modern scientific understanding.

In addition to personal experiences and cultural traditions, the book was also influenced by a growing body of scientific research supporting the efficacy of herbal medicine. Studies examining the pharmacological effects of plants, as well as their nutritional and therapeutic benefits, provided a solid foundation upon which to build the book's content. By grounding herbal remedies in evidence-based medicine, the author aimed to bridge the gap between ancient wisdom and contemporary healthcare practices.

Ultimately, "Herbal Remedies that Cure all Diseases" is a testament to the enduring power of nature to heal, nurture, and restore balance. It is a celebration of the remarkable synergy between humans and plants, and a call to rediscover the age-old wisdom that lies at the heart of herbal medicine.

READERS' TESTIMONIES

"Gabriel Olatuja's book profoundly deepened my spiritual journey. His insights on prayer and Christian growth are enlightening, guiding me to a closer relationship with God. A must-read for anyone seeking spiritual maturity and connection. Want to learn how to pray and get answers? Get Apostle's books on Amazon and you will not remain the same"
By Adetoun David-Mark, USA

"The Author's entrepreneurial wisdom is unparalleled. His book offers practical strategies and invaluable advice for navigating the complexities of business. A true game-changer, it's empowered me to thrive in the competitive world of entrepreneurship. Get his book on Amazon, you would be glad you did"
By Benny Lomeus, UK

"Apostle Gabriel-Wealth Olatuja's herbal remedies book is a treasure trove of natural healing. With his expertise, I've discovered effective solutions for various ailments, enhancing my well-being holistically. I'm changing the holistic approach to how I care for myself and my loved ones with these books."
By Sally Kole, Canada

ABOUT THE AUTHOR

Gabriel Olatuja is an Author and Publisher who has written books on entrepreneurship, Christian growth and effective prayers and motivational books, with thousands of copies sold world-wide. Gabriel is the founder of *Apostle Gabriel-Wealth Olatuja (AGO) Global Ministries* that blessed millions of people around the world. He is the publisher of *Apostle Gabriel-Wealth Olatuja Digital Library (APGODL)* with hundreds of free resources for daily living. He is a Pastor at Opulent Christian Assembly (City of Faith) Inc., Lagos, Nigeria. He is also a committed member of LoveWorld Inc.

Gabriel is the founder/CEO of Virtual Doctors Limited (www.virtualdoctors.ng) – a leading telemedicine company in Nigeria with over 5000 medical practitioners that provides digital healthcare to all Africans globally. He is also the Founder/CEO of Geewealth Technology – a software and technology consulting agency that has served thousands of business and individuals across in Africa, America, Canada, Europe and UAE. Gabriel also consults for local and international business in the area of technology deployment strategies and business development and marketing strategies. He has helped scores of business owners to start their business and helped push them to compete strongly across market landscapes.

Hear what he has to say about this book:

"Aside personal experience with the efficacy of roots and herbs in healthcare, I also got ancient knowledge from my grand-father's Herbal Book called "Apoti Imo" (Knowledge Box). The book contains the different herbal solutions to different ailments including cancer. I will be releasing these ancient live saving herbal

secrets in different volumes. Do not miss any of them." Gabriel-Olatuja

AUTHOR'S BOOKS

Some of the Author's best-selling books are
- Starting a Unicorn in Africa
- Raise up to $1 billion Dollar for your Startup
- Prayers That Work Supernatural Miracles
- Prayers for All Round Prosperity
- Mastering the Art of Equity and Investment
- 21 Days and Nights Effective Prayers For Supernatural Enlargement
- 100 Prayers to Opening the Floodgates of Financial Blessings

Several Copies of his books were sold with testimonies coming from readers. Get these books on Amazon at www.amazon.com/author/thebestsellingauthorx

DISCLAIMER

The information provided in this book, "Herbal Remedies that Cure all Diseases," is not a substitute for professional medical advice, diagnosis, or treatment.

Readers are advised to consult with a qualified healthcare professional before incorporating any herbal remedies or treatments mentioned in this book into their healthcare regimen, especially if they have underlying health conditions, are pregnant or nursing, or are taking medications. Readers can consult Medical Doctors at a fee on Virtual Doctors App.

The author and publisher of this book make no representations or warranties with respect to the accuracy, applicability, or completeness of the information provided. They shall not be held liable for any loss or damage arising from the use of the information contained in this book.

It is essential to exercise caution and discretion when using herbal remedies, as individual responses may vary. Always seek guidance from a healthcare professional to ensure safe and appropriate use of herbal remedies in conjunction with medical treatment.

By reading this book, you acknowledge that you have read, understood, and agreed to the terms of this disclaimer.

Copyright Protection Statement

INGREDIENTS SOURCING AND PREPARATION

For those facing challenges in sourcing or preparing the ingredients mentioned in the remedies, we offer a solution. Contact us to order raw or pre-prepared ingredients for a nominal fee. We ensure prompt delivery to your doorstep, no matter where you are located worldwide.

CONTACT

Email: gabrielolatuja@gmail.com, olatujagabriel@gmail.com
Call/WhatsApp: +2348067380225,
Website: www.gabrielolatuja.com.ng.

Table of Contents

REMEDY ONE - FEMALE FERTILITY BOOSTER

1.1 FEMALE FERTILITY

As a woman, experiencing challenges with fertility and facing difficulty getting pregnant can be an incredibly stressful and overwhelming journey. Despite the hardships of fertility struggles, it's important to recognize that you are not alone in this experience. Many individuals, much like yourself, encounter obstacles on the path to parenthood. According to the Mayo Clinic, 10-15% of couples grapple with infertility, defined as the inability to achieve pregnancy despite regular, unprotected intercourse for at least a year.

Given the widespread impact of infertility, various options are available to couples seeking assistance in conceiving. Assisted reproductive technologies, including in vitro fertilization (IVF), present viable solutions. However, it's crucial to acknowledge that IVF can be costly, invasive, and may not always yield success. If you are exploring alternative, more gentle, and natural methods to enhance fertility, you're not alone in that pursuit.

No matter the cause of your infertility, this naturally made fertility booster is so rich in nutrients, it can make you as a woman conceive by enhancing the production of eggs, reducing stress, decreasing inflammation, and increasing energy.

1.2 INGREDIENTS

1) Moringa leaves
2) Cinnamon Powder or sticks
3) Grounded cloves
4) Grounded fresh beet
5) Gorontula (ensure it's clean and prepared)
6) Honey
7) Water

1.3 NUTRITIONAL BENEFITS FOR BOOSTING FEMALE FERTILITY

1.3.1 Moringa

Moringa oleifera, commonly known as moringa, is recognized for its natural fertility-boosting nutrients. For those facing fertility challenges, moringa is believed to contribute to increased egg production, decreased inflammation, stress reduction, and enhanced energy levels.

As a nutrient-dense superfood, moringa may also play a role in balancing blood sugar levels and hormones, making it a valuable addition to fertility endeavors. Particularly, women dealing with PCOS may find moringa beneficial due to its insulin-mimicking proteins, potentially aiding in regulating insulin sensitivity and lowering blood sugar levels.

Moringa Leaves:

- Rich in essential vitamins and minerals, including vitamin A, vitamin C, calcium, and iron.
- High in antioxidants, which help combat oxidative stress and inflammation, contributing to reproductive health.
- Contains phytochemicals that may support hormonal balance.

1.3.2 Cinnamon Powder or Sticks

Cinnamon, whether in the form of powder or sticks, offers various nutrient compositions that can potentially contribute to boosting female fertility. Here are the key components and their potential benefits:

- **Antioxidants:** Cinnamaldehyde compound gives cinnamon its characteristic flavor and has antioxidant properties. Antioxidants help neutralize free radicals in the body, reducing oxidative stress, which can be beneficial for reproductive health.
- **Anti-Inflammatory Compounds:** Chronic inflammation can negatively impact fertility. Cinnamon contains Cinnamaldehyde and Cinnamic Acid which exhibit anti-inflammatory

properties, which may help reduce inflammation in the reproductive organs.

- **Regulation of Blood Sugar**: Cinnamon contains polyphenols that can enhance insulin sensitivity, helping to regulate blood sugar levels. Balanced blood sugar is essential for hormonal balance, which is crucial for fertility.
- **Trace Minerals:** Cinnamon is a good source of manganese, an essential trace mineral. Manganese plays a role in the synthesis of reproductive hormones and may support overall reproductive health.
- **Improved Circulation:** Cinnamon is a good source of cinnamaldehyde compound which may have vasodilatory effects, promoting improved blood circulation. Enhanced blood flow to the reproductive organs can be beneficial for fertility.
- **Aromatic Compounds:** Cinnamon contains essential oils with potential health benefits, including reproductive health. These oils may have positive effects on hormonal balance.
- **Aphrodisiac Properties:** Historical Beliefs Cinnamon has a long history of use as an aphrodisiac in various cultures. While scientific evidence is limited, the aromatic and warming

properties of cinnamon may have positive effects on mood and intimacy.

1.3.3 Grounded Cloves

Cloves, the aromatic flower buds of the clove tree (*Syzygium aromaticum*), are not only known for their distinctive flavor but also for their potential health benefits, including their role in supporting female fertility. The nutrient composition of cloves contributes to their positive effects on reproductive health:

- **Antioxidants:** Cloves are rich in antioxidants, particularly flavonoids, which help neutralize free radicals. This is crucial for protecting reproductive cells from oxidative stress, which can be a contributing factor to fertility issues.
- **Minerals:** Manganese: Cloves are an excellent source of manganese, an essential mineral that plays a role in the formation of reproductive hormones. Adequate manganese levels can contribute to hormonal balance, which is crucial for fertility.
- **Vitamin K:** Cloves contain vitamin K, which is important for blood clotting and may have positive effects on overall reproductive health.

- **Vitamin C:** This vitamin is known for its antioxidant properties and is important for immune function. It may also contribute to the health of the reproductive system.
- **Essential Oils:** Cloves contain essential oils, with eugenol being a prominent component. Eugenol has been studied for its potential anti-inflammatory and analgesic effects. Inflammation in the reproductive organs can negatively impact fertility, and the anti-inflammatory properties of eugenol may offer some benefits.
- **Nutrient Density:** Cloves are nutrient-dense, providing a range of essential nutrients in a small quantity. This includes trace amounts of other minerals such as iron, calcium, and magnesium, all of which play roles in various aspects of reproductive health.
- **Aphrodisiac Properties:** Traditionally, cloves have been associated with aphrodisiac properties, potentially influencing libido and sexual health. While more research is needed in this area, the historical use of cloves for enhancing reproductive function suggests a connection.

1.3.4 Grounded Fresh Beet

Beets, scientifically known as *Beta vulgaris*, are root vegetables that come in various vibrant colors, including deep red, golden, and white. These nutrient-rich vegetables offer a range of health benefits, and their nutrient composition makes them valuable for supporting female fertility. Here's an overview of the nutrient components found in beets that contribute to boosting female fertility:

- **Folate (Vitamin B9)**: Beets are a good source of folate, a crucial nutrient for reproductive health. Folate is essential for preventing neural tube defects during early pregnancy and supporting the development of the baby's neural tube.

- **Iron:** Iron is important for preventing anemia, a condition that can negatively impact fertility. Anemia can lead to reduced oxygen transport to reproductive organs, affecting their proper function.

- **Vitamin C:** Beets contain vitamin C, an antioxidant that helps protect cells from oxidative stress. Vitamin C is also known to enhance the absorption of non-heme iron (the type of iron found in plant-based foods like beets), further supporting iron metabolism.

- **Nitrate:** Beets are rich in dietary nitrates, which have been associated with improved blood flow. Enhanced blood flow can benefit reproductive health by ensuring that reproductive organs receive an adequate supply of oxygen and nutrients.
- **Potassium:** Potassium is essential for maintaining electrolyte balance and supporting proper muscle function. This is particularly relevant for the smooth muscles in the reproductive system.
- **Manganese:** Beets contain manganese, a trace mineral that plays a role in reproductive health. Manganese is involved in the synthesis of sex hormones and may contribute to hormonal balance.
- **Betaine:** Betaine is a compound found in beets that may have anti-inflammatory properties. Inflammation in the reproductive organs can negatively impact fertility, and betaine's anti-inflammatory effects may help alleviate this.
- **Dietary Fiber:** Beets are a good source of dietary fiber, which supports digestive health. Fiber helps regulate blood sugar levels and

may contribute to hormonal balance, both of which are important factors in fertility.

1.3.5 Gorontula

Although there is a limited scientific information about the effect of Gorontula (also known as "Snot Apple" or "Azanza Garckeana") on boosting female fertility, Gorontula is a tropical fruit native to West Africa and has been traditionally used in various cultures for its health benefits, including its potential to enhance fertility. Here are some general aspects and nutrients found in traditional medicine about this fruit that is relevant to boosting fertility:

- **Vitamins and Minerals:** Gorontula is believed to contain various vitamins and minerals essential for overall health, such as vitamin C and zinc. These nutrients play crucial roles in supporting reproductive functions.

- **Phytochemicals:** Like many fruits and plants, Gorontula contains phytochemicals. These plant compounds have antioxidant properties, helping to combat oxidative stress and protect reproductive cells from damage.

- **Aphrodisiac Properties:** In traditional medicine, Gorontula has been used as an aphrodisiac, suggesting a potential positive influence on libido and sexual function.

- **Hormonal Balance:** Some traditional practices associate Gorontula with promoting hormonal balance, which is crucial for regular menstrual cycles and overall reproductive health.
- **Nutrient Synergy:** The combination of nutrients in Gorontula may contribute to a synergistic effect, potentially providing comprehensive support for female fertility.

1.3.6 Honey

Honey is a natural sweetener that has been valued for its medicinal properties for centuries. Honey does offer a range of nutrients and health benefits that can contribute to overall well-being, which, in turn, may positively influence reproductive health. Here are some nutrient compositions and potential benefits of honey for boosting female fertility:

- **Antioxidants:** Honey is rich in antioxidants, including flavonoids and polyphenols. Antioxidants help neutralize free radicals in the body, reducing oxidative stress, which is crucial for maintaining a healthy reproductive system.

- **Energy Source:** Honey is a natural source of carbohydrates, primarily glucose and fructose. These sugars provide a quick and sustained energy boost, which is essential for supporting overall vitality and stamina, factors that are relevant to fertility.
- **Antibacterial and Anti-Inflammatory Properties:** Honey contains natural antibacterial properties, aiding in maintaining a healthy reproductive tract by preventing infections. The anti-inflammatory effects of honey may contribute to reducing inflammation in the reproductive organs, promoting a conducive environment for fertility.
- **Trace Elements:** Honey contains trace elements such as zinc, selenium, and copper, which are important for various physiological processes, including reproductive health. These elements play roles in hormone production and the maintenance of a healthy immune system.
- **Amino Acids:** Honey contains several amino acids, the building blocks of proteins. Amino acids are crucial for the synthesis of hormones

and enzymes, which are essential for reproductive processes.

- **Vitamins**: While not present in large amounts, honey does contain small amounts of vitamins, including vitamin C and some B vitamins. These vitamins play roles in immune function and energy metabolism, contributing indirectly to reproductive health.
- **Wound Healing and Tissue Repair:** Honey has been traditionally used for wound healing. While not directly related to fertility, the ability of honey to promote tissue repair may have implications for the health of the reproductive organs.
- **Digestive Health:** Honey may contribute to digestive health, aiding in nutrient absorption and ensuring that the body receives the necessary nutrients for overall well-being, including reproductive health.

1.4 PREPARATION INSTRUCTIONS

1.4.1 Combining the ingredients

- The combination of moringa, cinnamon, cloves, grounded fresh beet, gorontula, and honey provides a diverse range of nutrients that collectively support female fertility.

- Antioxidants from moringa, cinnamon, and cloves help protect reproductive cells from damage.
- Nutrients like iron, calcium, and folate from these ingredients contribute to overall reproductive health.
- Gorontula, with its traditional use, is believed to have specific benefits for female reproductive function.
- Honey adds natural sweetness and potential anti-inflammatory effects.

1.4.2 Measure Ingredients

- Use about 2 tablespoon of dried moringa leaves or 1 handful of fresh leaves.
- Add 2 cinnamon stick or 1 tablespoon of powdered cinnamon.
- Include 1 teaspoon of grounded cloves.
- Use about 2 tablespoon of grounded fresh beet root (adjust based on preference).
- Add a few pieces of Gorontula.
- Adjust honey to taste.

1.4.3 Combine Ingredients

- Place the measured moringa leaves, cinnamon stick, grounded cloves and Gorontula in a pot of 2 cups of water and boil for about 7 minutes. Put of the fire from the pot.
- Allow the mixture to steep for about 5-7 minutes. This lets the flavors infuse into the water.
- Add the grounded beet after steeping.

1.4.4 Strain

- After steeping, strain the tea to remove the leaves and other solid components. You can use a fine mesh strainer or a tea infuser.

1.4.5 Sweeten with Honey

- Add honey to the strained tea, adjusting the amount based on your sweetness preference.

1.4.6 Dosage

- Drink 1 cup in the morning and at night. You can store the remaining in the freezer for later use.

REMEDY TWO - GONORRHEA WITH BLOOD IN THE URINE (ATOSI ELEJE)

Gonorrhea, a sexually transmitted infection (STI) caused by the bacterium *Neisseria gonorrhoeae*, primarily affects the mucous membranes of the reproductive and urinary tracts. While gonorrhea itself may not directly lead to blood in the urine (hematuria), complications arising from untreated or poorly managed gonorrhea can potentially contribute to urinary symptoms, including hematuria. Here are some ways in which gonorrhea might indirectly lead to blood in the urine:

1. Urinary Tract Infection (UTI)

Gonorrhea can lead to infections in the urinary tract, including the urethra and bladder. These infections can cause inflammation and irritation of the urinary tract, which may result in symptoms such as pain during urination, frequent urination, and in some cases, hematuria.

2. Complications in Women

In women, untreated gonorrhea can spread to the reproductive organs, leading to pelvic inflammatory disease (PID). PID can cause inflammation and infection of the uterus, fallopian tubes, and ovaries. If the infection spreads to nearby structures, it may result in complications such as hematuria.

3. Complications in Men

Untreated gonorrhea in men can lead to epididymitis, which is inflammation of the epididymis—a coiled tube located at the back of the testicles. Epididymitis can cause pain, swelling, and potentially lead to complications such as hematuria.

2.1 INGREDIENTS

1) Christmas Melon (Tagiri fruit)
2) Bitter Melon
3) Potash
4) Azithromycin Tablet
5) Eftriaxone Tablet
6) Water

2.2 NUTRITIONAL BENEFITS

Let's explore the mentioned items and their components in curing atosi eleje:

2.2.1 Tagiri Fruit

- Tagiri fruit, also known as *Parkia biglobosa* or **African locust bean**, is commonly used in traditional medicine in the West African region.
- It contains various nutrients, including vitamins, minerals, and proteins.
- Some traditional beliefs suggest that Tagiri fruit may have anti-inflammatory properties, which could potentially be beneficial in addressing inflammation associated with hematuria.

2.2.2 Bitter Melon

- Bitter melon, also known as *Momordica charantia*, is a vegetable commonly used in traditional medicine for various health purposes.
- It is rich in antioxidants, including flavonoids and phenolic acids, which may have anti-inflammatory effects.
- Bitter melon is believed to have potential benefits for the urinary system, but scientific

evidence supporting its use for hematuria specifically is limited.

2.2.3 Potash

- Potash, also known as potassium carbonate, is an alkaline compound that has been historically used in traditional medicine for various purposes.
- Some traditional beliefs suggest that alkaline substances like potash may help balance the body's pH and reduce acidity, potentially benefiting the urinary system.
- However, the use of potash should be approached with caution, as excessive intake of alkaline substances can disrupt the body's acid-base balance and have adverse effects.

2.2.4 Azithromycin Tablets and Ceftriaxone Tablets

Azithromycin and ceftriaxone are commonly prescribed antibiotics for the treatment of gonorrhea, They help to enhance the effectiveness of treatment and to address potential strains of Neisseria gonorrhoeae that may be resistant to a single antibiotic.

2.3 PREPARATION INSTRUCTIONS

a) Cut 2-3 tagiri fruits into small pieces and put it in a container.
b) Cut 1 bara melon and put it in the same container.
c) Add some potash to the container
d) Ground 4 Tablets of Azithromycin and 4 Tablets of Ceftriaxone Tablets and add it to the container
e) Pour drinkable water inside the container.
f) Leave it for 2 days and start drinking from the 3rd day

2.4 DOSAGE

Drink one small cup in the morning and one in the evening.

REMEDY THREE - HYPERTENSION (EJE RIRU)

Hypertension, commonly referred to as high blood pressure, is a medical condition in which the force of blood against the walls of the arteries is consistently too high. It is a significant risk factor for various cardiovascular diseases and other health problems. Here are some key points about hypertension:

- Normal: Less than 120/80 mm Hg
- Elevated: 120-129/<80 mm Hg
- Hypertension Stage 1: 130-139/80-89 mm Hg
- Hypertension Stage 2: 140 or higher/90 or higher mm Hg
- Hypertensive Crisis: Higher than 180/120 mm Hg (emergency medical attention required)

Risk Factors: Several factors can contribute to hypertension, including genetics, age, diet, physical inactivity, excessive alcohol consumption, smoking, and certain medical conditions.

Complications: Untreated or poorly controlled hypertension can lead to serious health complications, such as heart disease, stroke, kidney damage, and eye problems.

1.2 INGREDIENTS
1. Two pieces of Alligator pepper
2. Tumeric (3 pieces)
3. Garlic (full of one hand)
4. Ginger (3 pieces)
5. 1 tablespoon of Lemon
6. A bottle of Pure honey

1.3 INGREDIENTS AND BENEFITS
1.3.1 Alligator Pepper
Alligator pepper, also known as grains of paradise or Aframomum melegueta, is a spice that is native to West Africa. It is commonly used in traditional medicine for various purposes, including potential benefits for cardiovascular health. However, it's important to note that while some studies suggest

certain health-promoting properties, the scientific evidence is not as extensive as with mainstream medications for high blood pressure. Here are some potential ways in which alligator pepper might be considered in relation to high blood pressure:

1. Anti-Inflammatory Properties

Alligator pepper contains bioactive compounds that may have anti-inflammatory effects. Chronic inflammation is linked to various cardiovascular conditions, including hypertension. By reducing inflammation, alligator pepper may contribute to overall heart health.

2. Antioxidant Effects

The spice is rich in antioxidants, which can help neutralize free radicals in the body. Antioxidants play a role in protecting blood vessels and preventing damage that could contribute to hypertension.

3. Vasodilatory Effects

Some studies suggest that Aframomum melegueta may have vasodilatory effects, meaning it may help relax blood vessels. This relaxation could potentially lead to improved blood flow and lower blood pressure.

4. Cardiometabolic Benefits

Alligator pepper may have effects on lipid metabolism and glucose regulation, which are factors associated with cardiovascular health. Improved management of these factors can indirectly contribute to the prevention or control of hypertension.

5. Diuretic Properties

Diuretics promote the excretion of excess salt and water from the body, potentially reducing blood volume and, consequently, blood pressure. Some herbs, including alligator pepper, are traditionally believed to have diuretic properties.

1.3.2 Ginger and Garlic

Both ginger and garlic have been studied for their potential benefits in promoting cardiovascular health, including the management of high blood pressure. Here's how ginger and garlic may contribute to the management of high blood pressure:

a. **<u>Ginger</u>**

Vasodilation: Ginger contains compounds like gingerol that may help promote vasodilation, the widening of blood vessels. This can contribute to improved blood flow and potentially help in lowering blood pressure.

Anti-Inflammatory Effects: Chronic inflammation may contribute to high blood pressure. Ginger has anti-inflammatory properties that may help reduce inflammation and support overall cardiovascular health.

Antioxidant Properties: Ginger is rich in antioxidants, which can help neutralize free radicals and reduce oxidative stress. Lowering oxidative stress is beneficial for maintaining healthy blood vessels.

b. <u>Garlic</u>

Allicin Content: Garlic contains allicin, a sulfur-containing compound with various health benefits. Allicin has been studied for its potential to relax blood vessels, which may contribute to lower blood pressure.

Antioxidant and Anti-Inflammatory Effects: Similar to ginger, garlic has antioxidant and anti-inflammatory properties that can help protect blood vessels and reduce inflammation, potentially supporting blood pressure regulation.

Improvement of Cholesterol Levels: Garlic has been associated with improvements in lipid profiles, including a reduction in LDL cholesterol levels. Managing cholesterol levels is essential for cardiovascular health and blood pressure regulation.

1.3.3 Turmeric

Contains curcumin, known for its anti-inflammatory and antioxidant properties. Turmeric may have cardiovascular benefits, including potential blood pressure regulation.

1.3.4 Lemon

Rich in vitamin C and antioxidants, lemon may help support heart health. It also contains compounds that may help lower blood pressure.

1.4 INSTRUCTIONS FOR PREPARATION

1. **Prepare the Ingredients**
   - Peel and clean the turmeric, garlic, and ginger.
   - Remove the seeds of the alligator pepper and ground the seeds to powder.

- Grind the turmeric and ginger into to fine particles.
- Grind the garlic for better infusion.
- Extract 2 tablespoons of lemon juice into a cup.

2. Combine Ingredients

- In a clean and dry glass or ceramic bowl, combine the grinded garlic, turmeric, ginger, alligator pepper and lemon juice and mix thoroughly.

3. Adding Honey

- Warm the honey slightly to make it more fluid. You can do this by placing the bottle in warm water, but avoid overheating to preserve the honey's beneficial properties.
- Slowly pour the warm honey into the herbal juice mixture, stirring continuously to ensure even mixing.

4. Bottling

- Once the honey and herbal mixture are well combined, carefully pour the herbal honey solution into a clean and dry glass or plastic bottle with a tight-sealing lid.

5. Storage

- Store the prepared herbal mixture in a cool, dark place to preserve its potency. Avoid direct sunlight, as it may affect the quality of the ingredients.
- Shake the bottle gently before each use to ensure that the herbal components are evenly distributed.

6. Usage and Dosage

- Adults can typically take 1 teaspoons of the herbal mixture in the morning and night daily.

REMEDY FOUR - MALE SPERM BOOSTER TEA

Infertility can be a significant concern for couples striving to conceive, and many individuals explore natural remedies to support reproductive health. Among the various options, certain ingredients have been traditionally associated with potential benefits for male sperm health. In this remedy, we will explore the nutritional benefits of a combination of natural ingredients known for their purported positive effects on male fertility. From the natural sweetness of honey to the rich compounds found in turmeric, moringa oleifera, bitter kola, ginger, cinnamon, basil (scent leaf), and dates, each ingredient brings a unique set of nutrients that may contribute to overall well-being, including potential support for sperm health.

1.5 NUTRITIONAL BENEFITS
1.5.1 Honey

- Nutritional Highlights: Rich in antioxidants, enzymes, and natural sugars.
- Potential Benefit: Antioxidants in honey may combat oxidative stress, promoting a healthier environment for sperm development.

1.5.2 Turmeric

- Nutritional Highlights: Contains curcumin, known for its anti-inflammatory and antioxidant properties.
- Potential Benefit: Curcumin may help reduce inflammation and oxidative stress, contributing to improved sperm quality.

1.5.3 Moringa Oleifera

- Nutritional Highlights: Packed with vitamins, minerals, and antioxidants.
- Potential Benefit: Nutrient density in moringa may support overall reproductive health and vitality.

1.5.4 Bitter Kola

- Nutritional Highlights: Contains caffeine, theobromine, and antioxidants.
- Potential Benefit: Traditionally believed to have aphrodisiac properties, bitter kola contributes to improved sexual function.

1.5.5 Ginger

- Nutritional Highlights: Contains gingerol with anti-inflammatory and antioxidant properties.
- Potential Benefit: Ginger may help reduce oxidative stress, promoting a favorable environment for sperm.

1.5.6 Cinnamon

- Nutritional Highlights: Rich in antioxidants, anti-inflammatory compounds, and minerals.
- Potential Benefit: Antioxidants in cinnamon may positively impact sperm health and motility.

4.1.7 Scent Leaf (Basil)

- Nutritional Highlights: Contains vitamins A and K, iron, and essential oils.

- Potential Benefit: Basil may contribute to overall reproductive health and hormonal balance.

1.5.7 Date
- Nutritional Highlights: High in natural sugars, fiber, and essential minerals.
- Potential Benefit: Dates provide energy and essential nutrients that may support reproductive well-being.

1.6 INGREDIENTS
1) 1 tablespoon honey (adjust to taste)
2) 1 teaspoon turmeric powder or a small piece of fresh turmeric
3) 1 teaspoon moringa oleifera powder or a handful of fresh leaves
4) 1 bitter kola nut, crushed
5) 1-inch piece of fresh ginger, sliced
6) 1 cinnamon stick
7) A handful of fresh basil (scent leaf) leaves
8) 1 date, pitted and chopped
9) 4 cups water

Note: You can scale up the amount of ingredient to achieve your desired quantity of the tea.

1.7 PREPARE INGREDIENTS

1. Wash and prepare all fresh ingredients, including turmeric, moringa leaves, ginger, basil leaves, and the date.
2. Boil Water - Bring 4 cups of water to a boil in a pot.
3. Add Ingredients to Boiling Water

Once the water is boiling, add the following ingredients to the pot and boil it for about 10 minutes:

- Turmeric powder or fresh turmeric
- Moringa oleifera powder or fresh leaves
- Crushed bitter kola
- Sliced ginger
- Cinnamon stick
- Chopped date

4. Add Basil (Scent Leaf): - Add the fresh scent leaves to the pot and simmer.
5. Simmer: - Reduce the heat to a simmer and let the ingredients infuse into the water for about 10-15 minutes.
6. Serving with Honey:- After a total simmering, take a cup of the tea, add 1-2 tablespoons of

honey and stir, adjusting the amount to your taste preference.

7. Optional Garnish: - If desired, you can garnish the tea with a fresh basil leaf or a slice of lemon.

8. Sip and enjoy your cup of multi-ingredient tea. Take a cup in the morning and at night.

Note: Warm the rest in the pot and serve the same way you did the first one. You tea pot can last for up to three days before preparing another one.

REMEDY FIVE - DIABETES MELITUS

Diabetes mellitus, commonly referred to as diabetes, is a chronic medical condition characterized by elevated levels of glucose (sugar) in the blood. There are different types of diabetes, with the two most common types being type 1 diabetes and type 2 diabetes. Here are some key points about diabetes:

5.0.1 Type 1 Diabetes

This is an autoimmune condition where the body's immune system mistakenly attacks and destroys the insulin-producing beta cells in the pancreas. People with type 1 diabetes must take insulin injections or use an insulin pump to replace the missing hormone. It often develops in childhood or early adulthood and is not related to lifestyle or diet.

5.0.2 Type 2 Diabetes

This is the most common form of diabetes and is often associated with lifestyle factors such as obesity, physical inactivity, and poor diet. In type 2 diabetes, the body either doesn't use insulin effectively (insulin resistance) or doesn't produce enough insulin. Management includes lifestyle changes (diet and exercise) and, in some cases, oral medications or insulin.

5.0.3 Symptoms

Common symptoms of diabetes include excessive thirst, frequent urination, unexplained weight loss, fatigue, blurred vision, slow-healing wounds, and increased susceptibility to infections.

5.0.4 Complications

Diabetes can lead to various complications if not well managed. These complications can affect the eyes (diabetic retinopathy), kidneys (diabetic nephropathy), nerves (diabetic neuropathy), and cardiovascular system (heart disease and stroke). Proper management of diabetes is crucial in preventing or delaying these complications.

5.1 INGREDIENTS

1. Bitter Melon (Ogiri Bara, Ogiri Bara, *Momordica charantia*)
2. African Mango (*Irvingia gabonensis*)
3. Cinnamon (*Cinnamomum verum*)
4. Ginger (*Zingiber officinale*)
5. Aloe Vera (*Aloe barbadensis miller*)
6. Neem (Dongoyaro, *Azadirachta indica*)
7. Scent Leaf (*Ocimum gratissimum*)
8. Bitter Leaf (Ewe Ewuro, *Vernonia amygdalina*)
9. Pawpaw (*Carica papaya*)
10. Drinking Water

5.2 INGREDIENTS AND BENEFITS

In Nigeria, traditional medicine often utilizes a variety of roots and herbs believed to have potential benefits for managing diabetes mellitus. Here are some roots and herbs that have been traditionally used in Nigeria for diabetes:

1. Bitter Melon (Ogiri Bara, *Momordica charantia*)

Bitter melon is a popular vegetable in Nigeria and is believed to have blood sugar-lowering properties. It is often consumed in various forms, including as a vegetable or as a juice.

2. African Mango (*Irvingia gabonensis*)

Also known as wild mango or bush mango, the seeds of the African mango are traditionally used in Nigeria and are believed to have potential benefits for managing diabetes.

3. Cinnamon (*Cinnamomum verum*)

Cinnamon is used as a spice in Nigerian cuisine and is believed to have anti-diabetic properties. It may help improve insulin sensitivity and regulate blood sugar levels.

4. Ginger (*Zingiber officinale*)

Ginger is a common spice in Nigerian cuisine, and it is believed to have anti-inflammatory and blood sugar-regulating properties. It can be consumed as a spice in cooking or as a tea.

5. Aloe Vera (*Aloe barbadensis miller*)

  - Aloe vera is used in traditional medicine and is believed to have potential benefits for diabetes. The gel extracted from the leaves may be consumed, but caution is advised due to potential side effects.

6. Neem (*Azadirachta indica*)

Neem leaves are traditionally used in Nigeria for various medicinal purposes, and they are believed to have anti-diabetic properties. Neem tea is a common form of consumption.

7. Scent Leaf (*Ocimum gratissimum*)

Scent leaf, also known as basil, is used in Nigerian cuisine and traditional medicine. It is believed to have anti-diabetic properties and is often used as a spice in cooking or consumed as a tea.

8. Bitter Leaf (*Vernonia amygdalina*)

Bitter leaf is traditionally used in Nigerian cuisine and is believed to have potential benefits for diabetes. It is often consumed as a vegetable or used in traditional concoctions.

9. Pawpaw (*Carica papaya*)

Pawpaw leaves are believed to have anti-diabetic properties and are used in traditional medicine. Pawpaw leaf tea is a common preparation.

5.3 INSTRUCTIONS FOR PREPARATION

1. Prepare the Ingredients

- Wash all fresh ingredients thoroughly.
- Cut the bitter melon into small pieces.
- Peel and cut the African mango into chunks.
- Grate or chop the ginger.
- Extract the gel from the aloe vera leaves, avoiding the yellow latex near the skin.

2. Boiling the Ingredients

1. Place bitter melon, African mango, cinnamon, ginger, aloe vera gel, neem leaves, scent leaf, bitter leaf, and pawpaw chunks in a large pot.
2. Add enough drinking water to cover the ingredients.

3. **Boil the Mixture**
    - Bring the mixture to a boil and then simmer over low heat.
    - Allow the mixture to simmer until the ingredients are well-cooked, and the water has reduced significantly.

4. **Straining the Mixture**
- Once the mixture has simmered and infused, strain the liquid to separate it from the solid parts. Use a fine strainer or cheesecloth to ensure a clear liquid.

5. **Cooling the Liquid**
- Allow the liquid to cool to room temperature.

6. **Storing the Traditional Medicine**
- Pour the cooled liquid into a clean, airtight container or bottle and store in a cool, dark place.

7. **Usage and Dosage**
- Consume the traditional medicine in moderation. Start with small amounts and monitor how your body responds.

REMEDY SIX - MALE AND FEMALE LIBIDO ENHANCER

Enhancing libido is a multifaceted aspect of sexual wellness, influenced by various factors, including physical, emotional, and nutritional elements. Several natural ingredients have been traditionally associated with potential benefits for both male and female libido. In this exploration, we delve into the nutritional compositions of selected ingredients known for their purported effects on libido enhancement.

1.8 NUTRITIONAL COMPOSITIONS
1.1 Hibiscus Plant (Zobo)
- Rich in antioxidants, including flavonoids.
- Contains vitamin C, iron, and other minerals.
- Potential benefits for blood circulation and overall cardiovascular health.

2. Turmeric
- Active compound curcumin has anti-inflammatory properties.
- May support blood flow and cardiovascular health.
- Antioxidant effects that may positively impact overall well-being.

3. Clove
- Contains eugenol, a compound with potential antioxidant and anti-inflammatory properties.
- May contribute to improved blood circulation.

4. Date

- High natural sugar content provides a quick energy boost.
- Rich in fiber, vitamins, and minerals.

5. Honey
- Natural sugars for energy.
- Contains antioxidants and enzymes.
- Potential benefits for overall health and vitality.

6. Ginger
- Gingerol, an active compound, may have anti-inflammatory effects.
- Supports blood circulation and cardiovascular health.

7. Garlic
- Contains allicin, known for potential cardiovascular benefits.
- May support blood flow.

8. Alcohol

- In moderation, alcohol may have relaxing effects.
- Excessive alcohol consumption, however, can have adverse effects on libido and overall health.

1.9 ALCOHOLIC LIBIDO ENHANCER PREPARATION

It's essential to drink responsibly and be mindful of individual health conditions.

1.10 INGREDIENTS

1. Hibiscus plant (Zobo) - 1 cups dried hibiscus petals
2. Turmeric - 1 tablespoon (powder or grated fresh)
3. Clove - 1 teaspoon (ground)
4. Date - 5 pieces (pitted and chopped)
5. Honey – 4 tablespoons
6. Ginger - 1 handful (chopped)
7. Cinnamon - 1 teaspoon (cinnamon stick preferable)
8. Garlic - 1 handful (chopped)
9. Alcohol

1.11 PREPARE OF INGREDIENTS

1. Ensure all ingredients are clean and properly prepared.
2. Add Hibiscus (Zobo) to 1 cup of drinkable water in the pot and boil for 5 minutes
3. Get a 1 bottle and add the boiled zobo(not with water), Turmeric, Clove, Date, Honey, Ginger, Cinnamon, Garlic to the 1 bottle
4. Add Alcohol - Once the ingredients have been packed into the bottle or container that has acover cover, fill the bottle or container with any quality Aromatic Schnnap or alcohol dry gin and cover it.
5. Store the bottle or container for at least3days to allow the useful components get extracted
6. Shake the bottle before drinking. Take 1 short (1 small cup) in the morning and at night.

REMEDY SEVEN - DIFFICULT CHILD BIRTH (DYSTOCIA)

Childbirth is a momentous event in a woman's life, as it can sometimes present challenges that hinder the natural process. When the normal course of labor encounters obstacles, it is termed "Dystocia." This remedy will remove the complexities of difficult childbirth and ensure the well-being of both mother and child during this transformative journey.

Disclaimer: *The information provided here is not medical advice and should not be considered a substitute for professional healthcare. This remedy for Dystocia is intended for informational purposes only. Always consult with qualified healthcare professionals for personalized guidance and care here.*

6.0 INGREDIENTS

- Jute Leaf (*Corchorus Olitorius*, **Ewedu** in Yoruba Language)

6.1 NUTRITIONAL COMPOSITIONS

Corchorus Olitorius (**Ewedu**): During childbirth, drinking juice extract from Corchorus olitorius, also known as jute leaf or ewedu by a woman in labour has been proven to enhance natural labor. While scientific evidence specifically linking jute leaf to childbirth is limited, its nutritional profile and sliming nature suggest potential advantages:

- **The Sliming Nature:** African traditional practices suggest that the slimy nature of jute leaf extract might be associated with potential benefits during labor. The slimy texture of jute leaf extract is thought to have lubricating properties, which some believe may help ease the passage of the baby through the birth canal. Additionally, it is suggested that the mucilaginous quality might provide a soothing effect, potentially reducing friction and discomfort during the birthing process.

- **Rich in Iron:** Jute leaf is a good source of iron, essential for preventing anemia during pregnancy and supporting overall maternal health.

- **Vitamin A Content:** The presence of vitamin A contributes to the development of the baby's eyes, skin, and immune system.
- **Folate Content:** Folate is crucial for the prevention of neural tube defects in the developing fetus.
- **Calcium Source:** Adequate calcium intake supports the development of the baby's bones and teeth.
- **Fiber Content:** Jute leaf is high in fiber, aiding in digestion and preventing constipation, common concerns during pregnancy.
- **Nutrient Variety:** Jute leaf contains various vitamins and minerals, contributing to a balanced and nutritious diet during pregnancy.

6.2 PREPARE OF INGREDIENTS

1) Get some of leaves of cochorus olitorus (Ewedu Vegetable).
2) Squeeze with hands into water or use blender to blend it into liquid form and mix it with water.
3) Extract the juice.

6.3 USAGE

1) The woman in labour should take one glass cup.
2) The baby will be delivered.

YORUBA: <u>FUN OBINRIN TO NROBI:</u> *E mu ewedu ki e si gbo sinu omi. E mu ife kan. E o si bi omo na ni irorun.*

CAUTION:
If a woman experiences difficulty giving birth and the situation persists after 30 minutes of using this remedy, it is imperative to seek immediate medical attention. Delaying professional medical assistance may pose risks to the well-being of both the mother and the child.

REMEDY EIGHT- NATURAL WAY OF SELECTING THE GENDER OF YOUR BABY

The two major factors that proven to be responsible for the gender are child are **the time of sexual intercourse** and **the lady's nutrition**. (*According to* <u>*National Library of Medicine*</u>)

The man plays a dominant role in selecting the sex of the child; having XY Chromosomes (both female and male respectively). The mother has XX Chromosomes.

The male sperm with Y chromosome are lighter in weight and swim faster than female ones, so they are more likely to reach the egg, but live short life. On the other hand, female sperm are heavier and live longer than male sperm.

Research work has shown that sex before ovulation may result in female child while sex during ovulation resulting in pregnancy is likely to produce a male child. So, if you have sex a few days before ovulation and then abstain (while the male sperm die), this would increase the chances of conceiving a girl.

Intercourse in the days before ovulation is recommended to have a daughter (a female child), and intercourse on the day of ovulation is recommended to have a son (a male child).

8.0 Exclusion criteria

People with the following should not bother to try the natural selection, they should consult gynaecologists. You can consult gynaecologist online at Virtual Doctors App - https://www.vvirtualdoctors.ng.

1. Illiterate women who could not follow orders
2. Men who had problems with spermogram disorder
3. Women who had high blood pressure
4. Women who had thyroid problems
5. Women who had neurological problems.
6. Women with secondary infertility.

8.2 NUTRITION

When a woman takes a combination of high sodium and potassium foods, it will increase the likelihood of having a male child.

On the other hand, when a woman takes a combination of foods with high calcium and magnesium, it will increase the likelihood of having a female child.

8.3. STEPS TO CONCEIVING A MALE CHILD

1. Time sex to coincide with the day of ovulation (no earlier than 24 hours before you are about to ovulate).
2. Deep penetrative sex is preferable. It helps if the woman orgasms.
3. Have an energy drink, a cup of coffee or some chocolate before having sex.

8.4.   STEPS TO CONCEIVING A FEMALE CHILD

1.1.1   Have intercourse within 2days (48hours) before ovulation and do not jave intercourse on your ovulation day.
1.1.2   Deep penetrative sex is preferable. It helps if the woman orgasms.

REMEDY NINE- SLEEPLESSNESS

Sleeplessness, or insomnia, is a prevalent condition affecting millions worldwide. It manifests in various forms, disrupting the natural sleep-wake cycle and impacting overall well-being. Understanding its causes, recognizing its symptoms, and seeking appropriate solutions are essential for managing this condition effectively.

Incorporating certain foods into your diet can not only boost blood levels but also promote better sleep quality. Fresh pumpkin leaves, natural honey, and milk are three such dietary components that offer a plethora of nutritional benefits, aiding in overall health and well-being. Let's delve into the specific advantages of each and how they can help address both blood level concerns and sleeplessness.

9.0.1 Causes of Sleeplessness

1. **Stress and Anxiety:** Excessive worry or stress can trigger insomnia by keeping the mind overly active, making it difficult to relax and fall asleep.
2. **Poor Sleep Habits:** Irregular sleep schedules, excessive screen time before bed, and consuming stimulants like caffeine late in the day can disrupt sleep patterns.
3. **Medical Conditions:** Certain medical conditions such as chronic pain, asthma, gastrointestinal issues, and hormonal imbalances can contribute to sleeplessness.
4. **Mental Health Disorders:** Conditions like depression, bipolar disorder, and post-traumatic stress disorder (PTSD) often coexist with insomnia, with each exacerbating the other.
5. **Medications:** Some medications, particularly those that affect neurotransmitters or hormones, can interfere with sleep patterns as a side effect.

6. **Environmental Factors:** Noisy environments, uncomfortable temperatures, and excessive light can disrupt sleep and contribute to insomnia.

7. **Lifestyle Choices:** Poor diet, lack of physical activity, and excessive alcohol or substance use can all negatively impact sleep quality.

9.0.2 Symptoms of Sleeplessness

1. **Difficulty Falling Asleep:** Individuals with insomnia often struggle to fall asleep, spending extended periods tossing and turning in bed.

2. **Frequent Awakenings:** Insomnia can cause frequent awakenings throughout the night, leading to fragmented sleep.

3. **Daytime Fatigue:** Despite spending time in bed, those with insomnia often wake up feeling tired and unrefreshed, leading to daytime fatigue and impaired cognitive function.

4. **Irritability and Mood Disturbances:** Sleeplessness can exacerbate irritability, mood swings, and difficulty managing emotions.

5. **Impaired Concentration and Memory:** Chronic sleeplessness can impair cognitive function, leading to difficulties with concentration, memory recall, and decision-making.

6. **Physical Symptoms:** Headaches, gastrointestinal disturbances, and muscle aches are common physical symptoms associated with chronic sleeplessness.

7. **Increased Risk of Chronic Health Conditions**: Prolonged insomnia is linked to an increased risk of developing chronic health conditions such as obesity, diabetes, and cardiovascular disease.

9.0.3 Lifestyle Solutions for Sleeplessness

1. Establish a Consistent Sleep Routine: Going to bed and waking up at the same time each day helps regulate the body's internal clock and promote better sleep.

2. Create a Relaxing Bedtime Routine: Engage in calming activities before bed, such as reading, listening to soothing music, or practicing relaxation techniques like deep breathing or meditation.

3. Optimize Sleep Environment: Ensure your bedroom is conducive to sleep by keeping it dark, quiet, and at a comfortable temperature.
4. Limit Stimulants and Electronics: Avoid caffeine and electronics (such as smartphones and computers) before bedtime, as they can interfere with the ability to fall asleep.
5. Address Underlying Medical Conditions: Consult with a healthcare professional to address any underlying medical or mental health conditions contributing to sleeplessness.

9.1 INGREDIENTS

1. Fresh Pumpkin Leaves, *Ewe Efo Ikoro (Yoruba), Ugwu Leave (Ibo)*
2. Natural Honey, *Oyin gidi (yoruba)*
3. Milk

9.2 NUTRITIONAL COMPOSITIONS AND BENEFITS

9.2.1 Fresh Pumpkin Leaves (Ewe Efo Ikoro/Ugwu Leaves)

- **Rich in Iron:** Fresh pumpkin leaves are a fantastic source of iron, a vital mineral essential for the production of hemoglobin in red blood cells. Adequate iron levels can prevent anemia, a condition characterized by low blood levels and fatigue.
- **High in Magnesium:** Magnesium, found abundantly in pumpkin leaves, plays a crucial role in regulating neurotransmitters that promote relaxation and sleep. It helps calm the nervous system, making it easier to fall asleep and stay asleep.
- **Loaded with Vitamins:** These leaves are packed with vitamins A, C, and E, which have antioxidant properties that support overall health and immune function, ensuring proper absorption of iron and other nutrients essential for blood health.

9.2.2 Natural Honey (Oyin Gidi)

- **Energy Boost:** Honey is a natural source of carbohydrates, providing a quick energy boost without causing a spike in blood sugar levels. Consuming honey before bedtime can help prevent nighttime awakenings due to hunger, promoting uninterrupted sleep.

- **Promotes Melatonin Production:** Honey contains tryptophan, an amino acid that stimulates the production of serotonin, which in turn converts into melatonin, the hormone that regulates the sleep-wake cycle. Consuming honey before bed may promote better sleep quality.
- **Supports Blood Health:** While not a direct source of iron, honey aids in the absorption of iron from other foods, thereby supporting healthy blood levels. Its antioxidant properties also protect red blood cells from damage.

9.2.3 Milk

- **Excellent Source of Calcium:** Milk is renowned for its calcium content, which is essential for maintaining strong bones and teeth. Calcium also plays a role in regulating the production of melatonin, promoting relaxation and improving sleep quality.

- **Contains Tryptophan:** Similar to honey, milk contains tryptophan, an amino acid precursor to serotonin and melatonin. Drinking a warm glass of milk before bedtime can have a calming effect on the nervous system, making it easier to fall asleep.
- **Hydration:** Staying hydrated is crucial for overall health, including sleep quality. Milk provides hydration along with its nutritional benefits, ensuring optimal bodily functions, including those related to sleep regulation.

9.3 PREPARATION INSTRUCTION

1. Wash the Fresh Pumpkin Leaves - Start by thoroughly washing the fresh pumpkin leaves under running water to remove any dirt or impurities.
2. Grind the Pumpkin Leaves – Grind the leaves into a liquid form.
3. Extract the juice - After grinding, carefully drain or use fine mesh to extra the juice from the shaft into a clean container.

4. Prepare the Milk – Add a tin of milk or dissolve powdered milk into water to taste. Pour the solution into the pumpkin juice.
5. Pour about 3-5 table spoonful of honey into the mixture and mix well.

9.4 DOSAGE/USAGE

Take a cup morning afternoon and night before bed. Take it for days until you have good sleep.

REMEDY TEN - VIRGINAL DISCHARGE

Vaginal discharge is a natural occurrence in women and serves as a vital function in maintaining vaginal health. However, changes in color, consistency, or odor of vaginal discharge may indicate underlying issues. Understanding the causes and symptoms of abnormal vaginal discharge is crucial for women's reproductive health.

Certain herbs and seeds have long been utilized in traditional medicine for their therapeutic properties, including their potential to address vaginal discharge issues. Clove, garlic, ginger, wonderful kola, and acacia seed are among the natural remedies known for their nutritional benefits in promoting vaginal health and combating infections. Let's explore their specific advantages:

10.1 CAUSES OF ABNORMAL VAGINAL DISCHARGE

1. Bacterial Vaginosis (BV) - BV occurs due to an imbalance of bacteria in the vagina, leading to an overgrowth of harmful bacteria. It often presents with a fishy odor and thin, grayish-white discharge.
2. Yeast Infection - Candida overgrowth, typically Candida albicans, causes yeast infections. Symptoms include thick, white, cottage cheese-like discharge accompanied by itching, redness, and irritation.

3. Sexually Transmitted Infections (STIs) - STIs such as gonorrhea, chlamydia, and trichomoniasis can cause changes in vaginal discharge. Discharge may be yellow, green, or frothy and often accompanied by other symptoms like itching, burning, or pain during urination or sex.
4. Pelvic Inflammatory Disease (PID) - PID is an infection of the female reproductive organs, often caused by untreated STIs. Symptoms include abnormal vaginal discharge, pelvic pain, fever, and painful intercourse.
5. Hormonal Changes - Fluctuations in hormone levels, such as those occurring during pregnancy, menstruation, or menopause, can alter vaginal discharge. Increased estrogen levels may lead to thicker, white discharge, while lower estrogen levels can result in less discharge.
6. Allergic Reactions or Irritation - Chemicals in soaps, douches, or feminine hygiene products can irritate the vagina, leading to changes in discharge. Allergic reactions to latex condoms or spermicides can also cause vaginal irritation and discharge.

10.2 SYMPTOMS OF ABNORMAL VAGINAL DISCHARGE

1. Changes in Color and Consistency

- o Discharge that is yellow, green, gray, or frothy in consistency may indicate an infection or STI.
- o Thick, white, clumpy discharge resembling cottage cheese is often a sign of a yeast infection.

2. Unpleasant Odor

- o A strong, fishy odor emanating from the vagina may indicate bacterial vaginosis or other infections.

3. Itching or Irritation

- o Persistent itching, burning, or irritation in the vaginal area, especially accompanied by abnormal discharge, suggests a potential infection or inflammation.

4. Pain or Discomfort

- o Pain during urination, intercourse, or pelvic discomfort may be indicative of underlying issues such as STIs or pelvic inflammatory disease.

5. Frequency and Duration

- o An increase in the frequency or duration of abnormal discharge, especially if accompanied by other symptoms, warrants medical evaluation.

10.3 INGREDIENTS

1. Clove
2. Garlic
3. Ginger
4. Wonderful Kola, *Buchholzia coriacea, Uke (Ibo), Uwuro (Yoruba), Ovu (Bini) Owi (Edo)*
5. Acacia Seed, *Bagaruwa (Hausa), Eso Booni (Yoruba)*

10.4 NUTRITIONAL COMPOSITIONS AND BENEFITS

1. Clove

- Antimicrobial Properties: Clove contains compounds like eugenol that exhibit potent antimicrobial properties, which can help

combat bacterial and fungal infections contributing to abnormal vaginal discharge.
- Anti-inflammatory Effects: Clove possesses anti-inflammatory properties that may help reduce inflammation and irritation in the vaginal area, alleviating discomfort associated with vaginal discharge issues.
- Rich in Antioxidants: The antioxidants found in cloves can help neutralize harmful free radicals and support overall immune function, aiding in the body's defense against infections.

2. Garlic

- Antibacterial and Antifungal Properties: Garlic contains allicin, a compound with strong antibacterial and antifungal properties, making it effective against various pathogens that may cause vaginal infections.
- Immune System Support: Garlic is rich in antioxidants and sulfur compounds that help strengthen the immune system, enhancing the body's ability to fight off infections and promote vaginal health.
- Anti-inflammatory Benefits: Garlic exhibits anti-inflammatory effects, which can help

reduce inflammation and irritation in the vaginal tissues, providing relief from discomfort associated with vaginal discharge issues.

3. Ginger

- Antioxidant and Anti-inflammatory Effects: Ginger contains bioactive compounds such as gingerol and shogaol, which possess antioxidant and anti-inflammatory properties that can help alleviate inflammation and support immune function.
- Digestive Health Support: Ginger aids in digestion and nutrient absorption, promoting overall gut health. A healthy gut microbiome is crucial for maintaining vaginal health and preventing infections.
- Circulation Improvement: Ginger has been shown to improve blood circulation, which may enhance nutrient delivery to the reproductive organs and support vaginal health.

4. Wonderful Kola (Buchholzia coriacea)

- Antimicrobial Properties: Wonderful kola exhibits antimicrobial activity against a range of pathogens, including bacteria and fungi, which can help combat infections contributing to vaginal discharge issues.
- Tonic Effect: Wonderful kola is traditionally used as a tonic to support overall health and well-being, including reproductive health.
- Potential Hormonal Balance: Some studies suggest that wonderful kola may have hormonal balancing effects, which could indirectly contribute to maintaining vaginal health.

5. Acacia Seed

- Astringent Properties: Acacia seed contains tannins with astringent properties that help tighten and tone mucous membranes, potentially reducing excessive vaginal discharge.
- Soothing Effect: Acacia seed is known for its soothing properties, which can help alleviate irritation and discomfort associated with vaginal discharge issues.
- Nutrient-Rich: Acacia seed is a good source of nutrients such as vitamins, minerals, and

dietary fiber, which support overall health and may contribute to vaginal health.

10.5   PREPARATION INSTRUCTION
1. Soaking Clove

- Take a handful of cloves and thoroughly wash them using clean water to remove any dirt or impurities.
- Place the washed cloves in a clean container or bowl with cover.
- Fill the container with enough water to completely submerge the cloves.
- Cover the container with a lid or cloth to prevent dust or insects from getting in.
- Allow the cloves to soak in water for three days at room temperature. This soaking process helps extract the beneficial compounds from the cloves.
- **USAGE:** Use the clove extract as a vaginal wash or douche once or twice a day, depending on the severity of the vaginal discharge issues.

2. Boiling Garlic, Ginger, Wonderful Kola, and Acacia Seed

- Peel and crush a few cloves of garlic to release their medicinal properties.
- Peel and slice a piece of fresh ginger root into smaller pieces.
- Wash the Wonderful Kola and Acacia Seed thoroughly to remove any debris.
- In a clean pot, add enough water to cover all the ingredients.
- Add the crushed garlic, sliced ginger, washed Wonderful Kola, and Acacia Seed to the pot of water.
- Bring the water to a boil over medium heat.
- Once the water starts boiling, reduce the heat and let the mixture simmer for about 25-40 minutes. This allows the herbs and seeds to infuse their beneficial properties into the water.
- After simmering, remove the pot from the heat and allow the mixture to cool down to a comfortable temperature.

3. Straining the Herbal Solution

- Once the herbal mixture has cooled, strain it through a fine mesh sieve or cheesecloth to remove any solid particles.

- Transfer the strained herbal solution into a clean glass container or bottle. Discard the leftover solids.

-

10.6 DOSAGE/USAGE

- Store the herbal solution in the refrigerator to keep it fresh.
- To use, take a small amount of the herbal solution and dilute it with warm water if desired.
- It's essential to perform a patch test before using the herbal solution extensively to ensure there are no allergic reactions or irritations.

Constipation is a common gastrointestinal issue characterized by infrequent bowel movements or difficulty passing stools. It can vary in severity and duration, impacting individuals of all ages. Understanding the causes and symptoms of constipation is essential for proper management and prevention.

11.0.1 Causes of Constipation

1. Dietary Factors

- Low Fiber Intake: Diets low in fiber, such as those high in processed foods and low in fruits, vegetables, and whole grains, can contribute to constipation.

- Inadequate Fluid Intake: Dehydration can lead to hard, dry stools that are difficult to pass, resulting in constipation.

2. Lifestyle Choices

- Lack of Physical Activity: Sedentary lifestyles and lack of regular physical activity can slow down the digestive system, contributing to constipation.
- Ignoring the Urge to Defecate: Ignoring the natural urge to have a bowel movement can lead to stool retention and constipation over time.

3. Medications

- Certain medications, including opioids, antacids containing aluminum or calcium, antidepressants, and iron supplements, can cause constipation as a side effect.

4. Medical Conditions

- Irritable Bowel Syndrome (IBS): Individuals with IBS may experience constipation as one of the symptoms, along with abdominal pain and bloating.

- Hypothyroidism: Underactive thyroid function can slow down metabolism and digestive processes, leading to constipation.
- Colorectal Disorders: Conditions such as anal fissures, hemorrhoids, and colorectal cancer can cause pain and discomfort during bowel movements, leading to constipation.

5. Neurological Disorders

- Conditions that affect the nerves controlling bowel movements, such as multiple sclerosis (MS) or Parkinson's disease, can result in constipation.

11.0.2 Symptoms of Constipation

1. Infrequent Bowel Movements - Bowel movements occurring less than three times per week may indicate constipation.
2. Difficulty Passing Stools - Straining during bowel movements or feeling like the stool

is hard, dry, or incomplete can be symptoms of constipation.

3. Abdominal Discomfort - Abdominal bloating, cramping, or discomfort may accompany constipation, especially when there is stool buildup in the intestines.
4. Rectal Bleeding - Straining during bowel movements can cause small tears in the skin around the anus, leading to rectal bleeding, particularly in cases of chronic constipation.
5. Sensation of Incomplete Evacuation - Feeling like there is still stool left in the rectum after a bowel movement is a common symptom of constipation.
6. Changes in Stool Consistency - Stools that are hard, dry, lumpy, or difficult to pass are indicative of constipation.
7. General Discomfort and Fatigue - Chronic constipation can cause general discomfort, fatigue, and a sense of unease, impacting overall well-being.

11.1 INGREDIENTS

1. Bitter melon (fresh or dried)

2. Bitter kola nuts
3. Cashew bark (fresh or dried)
4. Alcohol (such as Schnapps, vodka or brandy)

11.2 NUTRITIONAL COMPOSITIONS AND BENEFITS

1. Bitter Melon

- Rich in Fiber: Bitter melon is a good source of dietary fiber, which adds bulk to stool and promotes regular bowel movements. Adequate fiber intake is essential for preventing and relieving constipation.
- Antioxidant Properties: Bitter melon contains antioxidants such as vitamin C, vitamin A, and flavonoids, which help reduce inflammation in the digestive tract and support overall gastrointestinal health.

2. Bitter Kola

- Digestive Aid: Bitter kola contains compounds that stimulate the production of gastric juices and promote digestion. Improved digestion can contribute to regular bowel movements and alleviate constipation.

- Anti-inflammatory Effects: Bitter kola possesses anti-inflammatory properties that may help reduce inflammation in the digestive system, potentially easing symptoms of constipation.

3. Cashew Bark

- Mild Laxative Properties: Cashew bark is traditionally used in some cultures as a natural remedy for digestive issues, including constipation. It is believed to have mild laxative effects that can help stimulate bowel movements.
- Antimicrobial Benefits: Cashew bark contains certain compounds that exhibit antimicrobial properties, which may help maintain a healthy balance of gut bacteria and support optimal digestive function.
-

11.3 PREPARATION INSTRUCTION
1. Preparation of Ingredients

- Wash the bitter melon thoroughly in water to remove any dirt or impurities. If using dried bitter melon, ensure it is clean and free from contaminants.
- Slice it bitter kola nuts into smaller pieces. For dried bitter melon, crush or grind or slice it into smaller pieces using a mortar and pestle, knife or a food processor.
- Measure out the desired amount of cashew bark. If using dried bark, crush it into smaller pieces to increase surface area and aid in extraction.

2. Combining Ingredients

- Place the prepared bitter melon, bitter kola nuts, and cashew bark into a clean jar bottle or container.
- Pour enough alcohol over the ingredients to fully cover them. Ensure that the alcohol completely submerges the plant materials.

3. Sealing and Storage

- Secure the lid tightly on the container or bottle to prevent any leakage or evaporation.

- Store it in a cool, dark place away from direct sunlight. Allow the mixture to steep for at least 3-5 days to extract the beneficial compounds from the ingredients. Shake the jar gently every few days to agitate the contents.

DOSAGE/USAGE

- Store the bottle/container in a cool, dark place until ready to use.
- Take one glass cup morning and night

Always consult with a qualified healthcare provider before using herbal remedies, especially if you have underlying health conditions or are taking medications.

DEDICATION

This book is dedicated to those who have suffered due to inefficient medical practices, those who have lost their lives and those who have endured the adverse effects of medications and vaccines.

AKNOWLEDGEMENT

I extend my heartfelt gratitude to my beloved wife, Orobola Olatuja-Gabriel, whose unwavering support and encouragement were instrumental in the compilation of this book.

I pay tribute to my esteemed late grandfather, Olatuja Adeyankinnu, whose life's work in herbal medicine, notably encapsulated in the timeless tome "Apoti Imo" (Knowledge Box), continues to inspire and guide my own journey.

Special thanks are also due to my late father, Martins Aregbesola Olatuja, whose dedication to preserving our family's herbal healing legacy ensures that this invaluable knowledge remains accessible to future generations.

May their wisdom, passion, and legacy infuse these pages, enriching the lives of readers seeking natural paths to health and well-being.